THE SIMPLE WALL PILATES EXERCISES FOR BEGINNERS

A step by step training guide to Gain Flexibility, Strength and Balance

Contents

How It Got Started.. 5

Chapter 1... 6

The Basics.. 6

The Importance Of Wall Pilates.. 9

The Different Between Wall Pilates And Traditional Pilates.................................... 11

Chapter 2... 12

How You Can Set Up Workout Space.. 12

Setting Up a Pilates-Friendly Environment.. 13

The Important Equipment for Wall Pilates.. 15

Safety Considerations... 17

Chapter 3... 19

The Foundational Wall Pilates Exercises.. 19

The Gentle Warm-Up Movements... 22

Core-Strengthening Techniques.. 23

Leg and Arm Exercises for Beginners...26

Chapter 4... 28

Building Strength and Flexibility...28

Progressive Exercises for Muscle Endurance..30

Stretching Into Wall Pilates.. 32

Adapting Movements to Your Fitness Level.. 34

Chapter 5... 36

Create Your Wall Pilates Routine.. 36

How To Design a Personalized Workout Plan..40

Combining Exercises for Full-Body Engagement.. 41

My Secret for Consistency and Progress Tracking...42

Chapter 6... 44

The Advanced wall Pilate Exercises.. 44

Wall Push up Work.. 44

Single Leg Wall Bridge.. 46

Wall Plank.. 48

Wall Pick.. 49

Wall Abdominal Curl..50

Chapter 7... 51

5 Simple Practical EXERCISES.. 51

ONE-SIDED WALL SLIDING... 51

GLUTE BRIDGE TO THE WALL... 52

LATERAL EXTENSION TO THE WALL... 53

ANGEL ON THE WALL...**54**

THUMB TO THE WALL..**55**

Bonus...**57**

Practical Videos Workout...**57**

28 Days Workout Challenge Plan..**58**

Conclusion...**62**

How It Got Started

Meet Bryan Wilson, a 64-year-old carpenter and musician whose journey with Pilates defies the clichés and exceeds expectations. Before embracing Pilates, Bryan's days were filled with physical labor and musical performances, each activity straining his body in distinct ways. Despite the strain, Bryan eschewed Pilates for nearly two decades, suspicious of its relevance to his busy lifestyle. Yet, chronic agony and a need for relief finally drove him to reconsider.

Initially, Bryan's hopes were modest—he hoped for some relief from his persistent back pain and greater mobility. But Pilates offered him far more than he thought. Gradually, through individualized training and continuous practice, Bryan discovered a greater power and agility he never believed possible. As his muscles changed and his motions grew more fluid, the once-skeptical carpenter found himself moving with increased confidence and ease.

What sets Pilates different for Bryan is its precision and attention to technique. Unlike standard weightlifting regimens, Pilates stresses regulated movements and core activation, leading to leaner, more functioning muscles. Bryan's metamorphosis wasn't simply physical; it was a comprehensive one that improved his complete well-being. Gone were the days of scheming to avoid harm; instead, he embraced movement with a fresh freedom and delight.

Reflecting on his path, Bryan notes the initial difficulty of adapting to Pilates' synchronized movements and focusing on core activation. Yet, those problems were overshadowed by the actual benefits he experienced—increased strength, movement, and a great sense of life. Pilates, once regarded as "not for him," became a key element of Bryan's regimen, offering him a road to longevity and vigor in his demanding work and passion for music.

For those apprehensive to attempt Pilates, Bryan offers words of encouragement. Whether you're handling a physically demanding profession or simply seeking to move with greater ease, Pilates may be transformative. It's not about fast outcomes but rather a journey of discovery and growth. With patience and determination, you'll unleash your body's full potential and rediscover the joy

of movement. So, why wait? Take the first step towards a healthier, more vibrant self with Pilates

Chapter 1

The Basics

Pilates is a low-impact exercise regimen that aims to improve muscle strength, flexibility, and posture. Exercises usually last 45 to an hour and take place in a classroom setting. You move slowly and deliberately, matching your movements to your breathing.
Although the primary focus will be on your core muscles, you may also target your arms, glutes, and lower legs.

So, what exactly is wall pilates?
Wall pilates is a variation that engages your muscles and improves flexibility by using a wall as resistance and your own body weight.
Unlike traditional pilates, this method does not require any specialized equipment. Wall stability gives support while you gently and methodically stretch and tone your muscles.

How Effective is Wall Pilates?
An added layer of resistance from the wall improves stability and promotes muscle growth.
It's especially useful for novices because it promotes stability and makes it easier to achieve difficult positions.

Warm-up Wall Pilates Routine: Compliant Move on.
Take a proud stance against the wall, back to it.
Step backward so that your feet are six inches apart.
Tension your core while maintaining a comfortable, downcast posture.
After taking a deep breath, gently glide your spine down the wall, vertebra by vertebra.
As you sink, feel your back muscles stretch.
As you approach the bottom of the roll, release the air while keeping your arms at your sides.
Hold for a few breaths.
Inhale as you raise yourself back to the beginning position. Repeat five more times.

Open the hips higher.
Stand close to the wall and place one hand on it for support.
Raise your outside leg till your thigh reaches the ground.
Maintain a forward stance with a level pelvis.
Put your inside hand on your lifted thigh for support.
Breathe out, stretch your leg out to the side, and gently place it on your hand.
Hold for a few breaths.

Inhale, then release your leg to return to the beginning position. Proceed to the opposite side.

Lateral swing of the legs
Stand close to the wall and place one hand on it for support.
Raise your outside leg till your thigh reaches the ground.
Maintain a forward stance with a level pelvis. Swing your leg out to the side and as high as possible, maintaining your pelvis level.
Swing your leg in the other direction to get back to the starting position.
Proceed to the opposite side.

Intensive Extension of the Calf
As you stand near the wall, place your palms flat against it at shoulder height.
Step back with your left leg for roughly two feet, keeping your heel flat on the floor.
Bend your right knee and lean against the wall until your left calf begins to stretch. Keep your left leg straight.
Hold for a few breaths.
Let go and repeat on the opposite side.

Main Workout (2 Circuits): Suitable Parts Lean
Stand close to the wall and place one hand on it for support.
Lean your left leg back a few steps and place your left hand flat against the wall.
Flex your right knee, lean your chest forward, and keep your heel down while stretching your left hamstring.
Hold for a few breaths. Let go and repeat on the opposite side.

Stand with your knees lifted.
Stand close to the wall and place one hand on it for support.
Keep your core firm and lift your right knee to your chest.
Tuck your lower back against the wall and elevate your knees.
Hold for a few breaths. Let go and repeat on the opposite side.

Wall with DB Arm Raise
Assume a wall stance, holding a light dumbbell in each hand with your elbows bent 90 degrees.
Tighten your core and gradually raise your arms until they are parallel to the ground.
After a few breaths of holding, return your arms to their initial position.
DB Arm Circles Walls
Stand against the wall with your elbows bent 90 degrees and a light dumbbell in each hand.
Tighten your core as you progressively bring your arms parallel with the floor.
Make small circular motions in the air for thirty seconds before changing course and repeating for another thirty seconds.

Torso extenders
Stand with your back to the wall, feet about two feet apart.
Place your hands shoulder-height on the wall, flat.
Tense your abs and push your chest into the wall as you slide your hands up to fully extend your arms overhead.
After a few breaths of holding, return to the starting posture.

Recess Walls
Stand with your back to the wall, feet about two feet apart.
When your thighs are parallel to the floor, carefully down the wall.
Maintain this pose for as long as possible, or at least 30 seconds.

Cool down: Take a seat across from the toe tap.
Begin by sitting on the floor, legs out in front of you, back against the wall.
When you spread your legs, they should be around hip width apart.
Press your lower back against the wall while tensing your ab muscles.
From this point, stretch your left hand and tap your right toes.
Switch sides for 45 seconds, or whatever long you can.

Chair-Side Spine Twist
Begin by sitting on the floor, legs out in front of you, back against the wall.
When you spread your legs, they should be around hip width apart.
Make your abs tighter.
From this position, stretch your left hand to touch the floor outside of your right leg and rotate your torso to the right.
Turn the twist around and bring your right hand to the floor past your left leg.
Switch sides for 45 seconds, or whatever long you can.

Butterfly Extend
Take a sit on the floor with your back to the wall and your legs bent in front of you, bringing the soles of your feet together.
Press your low back into the wall and let your knees drop to the sides.
Arch your back away from the wall and raise your arms above this position.
After a few breaths of holding, return to the starting posture.

Forward-seated fold.
Take a sit on the floor with your back to the wall and your legs bent in front of you, bringing the soles of your feet together.
Press your low back into the wall and let your knees drop to the sides.

From this position, raise your arms overhead and lean forward at the hips, allowing your shoulders and head to hang heavy.
After a few breaths of holding, return to the starting posture.

Wall pilates, which does not require expensive equipment, is a wonderful way to boost your exercise regimen. It's a basic at-home core workout that everyone can do, regardless of experience level, back discomfort, or other issues. Try it out and see the benefits for yourself.

The Importance Of Wall Pilates

Pilates is a low-impact exercise regimen that aims to improve muscle strength, flexibility, and posture. Exercises usually last 45 to an hour and take place in a classroom setting. You move slowly and deliberately, matching your movements to your breathing.
Although the primary focus will be on your core muscles, you may also target your arms, glutes, and lower legs.

So, what exactly is wall pilates?
Wall pilates is a variation that engages your muscles and improves flexibility by using a wall as resistance and your own body weight.
Unlike traditional pilates, this method does not require any specialized equipment. Wall stability gives support while you gently and methodically stretch and tone your muscles.

How Effective is Wall Pilates?
An added layer of resistance from the wall improves stability and promotes muscle growth.
It's especially useful for novices because it promotes stability and makes it easier to achieve difficult positions.

Warm-up Wall Pilates Routine: Compliant Move on.
Take a proud stance against the wall, back to it.
Step backward so that your feet are six inches apart.
Tension your core while maintaining a comfortable, downcast posture.
After taking a deep breath, gently glide your spine down the wall, vertebra by vertebra.
As you sink, feel your back muscles stretch.
As you approach the bottom of the roll, release the air while keeping your arms at your sides.
Hold for a few breaths.
Inhale as you raise yourself back to the beginning position. Repeat five more times.

Open the hips higher.
Stand close to the wall and place one hand on it for support.

Raise your outside leg till your thigh reaches the ground.
Maintain a forward stance with a level pelvis.
Put your inside hand on your lifted thigh for support.
Breathe out, stretch your leg out to the side, and gently place it on your hand.
Hold for a few breaths.
Inhale, then release your leg to return to the beginning position. Proceed to the opposite side.

Lateral swing of the legs
Stand close to the wall and place one hand on it for support.
Raise your outside leg till your thigh reaches the ground.
Maintain a forward stance with a level pelvis. Swing your leg out to the side and as high as possible, maintaining your pelvis level.
Swing your leg in the other direction to get back to the starting position.
Proceed to the opposite side.

Intensive Extension of the Calf
As you stand near the wall, place your palms flat against it at shoulder height.
Step back with your left leg for roughly two feet, keeping your heel flat on the floor.
Bend your right knee and lean against the wall until your left calf begins to stretch. Keep your left leg straight.
Hold for a few breaths.
Let go and repeat on the opposite side.

Main Workout (2 Circuits): Suitable Parts Lean
Stand close to the wall and place one hand on it for support.
Lean your left leg back a few steps and place your left hand flat against the wall.
Flex your right knee, lean your chest forward, and keep your heel down while stretching your left hamstring.
Hold for a few breaths. Let go and repeat on the opposite side.

Stand with your knees lifted.
Stand close to the wall and place one hand on it for support.
Keep your core firm and lift your right knee to your chest.
Tuck your lower back against the wall and elevate your knees.
Hold for a few breaths. Let go and repeat on the opposite side.

Wall with DB Arm Raise
Assume a wall stance, holding a light dumbbell in each hand with your elbows bent 90 degrees.
Tighten your core and gradually raise your arms until they are parallel to the ground.
After a few breaths of holding, return your arms to their initial position.

The Different Between Wall Pilates And Traditional Pilates

A variation of classical Pilates known as wall Pilates uses a wall to provide resistance and support. Wall Pilates exercises are performed with the body pressed against the wall, adding an extra aspect to the workout. Compared to traditional Pilates movements performed on a mat or with specialized equipment, this can increase muscle stability, alignment, and engagement. The wall is an effective tool for refining motions and providing additional feedback for proper posture and form.

Pilates on the wall: Using the wall adds a new dimension to the routines. Compared to regular Pilates, there are some notable modifications and benefits:

Wall Pilates uses the wall to provide stability and support for a variety of actions, promoting consistency and efficiency. This could be especially useful for people who are just starting off or attempting to become more steady.

The wall guides proper posture and alignment. It helps users maintain good posture while working out, ensuring that motions are completed correctly and the relevant muscle groups are engaged.

Wall Pilates can increase the intensity of some moves by employing the wall as resistance. Compared to traditional Pilates, the resistance from the wall forces individuals to gain strength and control in a novel way by working muscles in different ways.

Variety of Movements: Wall Pilates expands the range of possible movements. Participants can choose from a range of exercises that employ the wall for additional variations, making the workout more dynamic and exciting.

Improved Mind-Body Connection: The wall acts as a tactile signal, strengthening the mind-body connection. Participants may feel the wall's support and resistance, which increases their awareness of their actions and muscular activation.

Accessible for a Wide Range of Fitness Levels: The wall can make Pilates more accessible to those with various levels of fitness or particular medical needs. It allows for changes to fit the needs and capabilities of each individual.

Wall Pilates allows for specific muscle activation. The wall helps participants isolate their muscles, allowing them to focus on precisely training and strengthening those particular body parts.

Therapeutic Benefits: Wall Pilates is an excellent alternative for anyone with special diseases or physical restrictions due to the potential therapeutic benefits of the wall's support. It gives additional support and allows for more controlled movements.

Wall Pilates, which use the wall as a valuable tool for improving stability, alignment, and resistance in the pursuit of a balanced and strengthened body, is an innovative and successful variation on traditional Pilate.

Chapter 2

How You Can Set Up Workout Space

Setting up a room for Pilates, whether Wall Pilates or normal Pilates, requires making it safe, comfortable, and conducive to focus and movement. To help you put up a decent Pilates area, consider the following steps:

Empty the Space

Clear any debris or barriers from the designated Pilates area. Make sure you have enough space for your workouts so you can walk around freely without bumping into any furniture or other objects.

Employ a mat or padding: When performing Pilates on the floor, use a mat or a padded surface to provide comfort. This keeps your body cushioned and helps you retain stability while doing out.

Proper lighting.

Make sure the space is well-lit to create a cheerful and friendly atmosphere. Natural light is desirable, although artificial lighting that adequately illuminates the space can be utilized in its place.

Ventilation: To keep the air clean when working out, choose an area with good ventilation. It is critical to maintain enough ventilation, especially when engaging in activities that may increase your breathing and heart rate.

Calm Ambience: Choose a peaceful environment to reduce disturbances. Turn off all electronics and notifications so you can fully concentrate on your Pilates exercise.

Mirror (optional). If you're doing routines that need precise alignment, consider placing a mirror in the area. A mirror allows you to visually assess good form and posture.

Props & Equipment: Make sure you always have access to any props or equipment you might require for your Pilates practice. This could include stability balls, resistance bands, or any other specialty equipment required for the activities you've chosen.

Adorable Clothing:

Put on loose, breezy clothing that will not limit your range of motion. This enhances your overall comfort level and makes it easier to do Pilates routines correctly.

Bare feet or grippy socks: Shoes are not always required when performing Pilates. If you're practicing on a mat, you should wear grippy socks or go barefoot to maintain stability and prevent slipping.

Mindful Ambiance: Consider creating a quiet space or playing relaxing music to promote a mindful environment. This may make your Pilates practice more enjoyable and stress-free.

Keep in mind that the secret is to create an environment that encourages constant practice and keeps you motivated. Adapting these guidelines to your preferences will help you establish a productive and encouraging Pilates environment.

Setting Up a Pilates-Friendly Environment

Creating a place that adheres to Pilates principles is part of establishing a Pilates-friendly environment that allows for targeted and effective exercises. This is a guide to help you create a pleasant Pilates space:

Choose a venue or room with adequate space for your Pilates activities. Make sure there are no obstructions in the way of your arms and legs as they expand.

Light from nature:

If at all possible, use natural lighting. It improves your entire Pilates experience by creating a positive and energetic environment.

Pleasant Flooring:

A mat or comfortable flooring can provide enough support when conducting floor workouts. This is especially important for occupations that involve kneeling or lying down.

Arrangement in order:

Organize your Pilates props and equipment. This keeps your workout environment organized and makes it easy to find everything you need.

Mirrors For Input:

When working out, consider strategically situating mirrors to ensure proper alignment and form. Mirrors are important for assessing technique and making required adjustments.

Props and Stability Balls:

Make sure you always have access to your stability ball, resistance bands, and any other Pilates props you use. This allows for a smooth transition between exercises.

Calm Ambience:

Reduce outside noise to create a peaceful and attentive environment. This can include choosing a tranquil environment or playing soothing background music.

Getting air:

When working out, ensure that there is adequate ventilation to keep the air clean. Good ventilation helps to create a welcome and comfortable workout environment.

Consistent colors:

Consider designing your Pilates studio in muted shades. A peaceful environment with neutral hues can promote concentration and serenity.

Concise Design

Include items in your space that inspire mindfulness, such as artwork or plants. Encouraging decor or a touch of nature can improve the atmosphere for working out.

Electronic detox:

Set aside a part of your Pilates studio with no electronics. This allows you to avoid outside distractions and focus solely on your breathing and motions.

Temperature Management:

Keep your Pilates area at a reasonable temperature. To ensure that you can move freely during your workout, avoid getting too hot or too cold.

Remember that the goal is to create a space during your Pilates workouts that promotes focus, ease, and engagement. Modify these guidelines to suit your preferences and create a Pilates room that is uniquely yours.

The Important Equipment for Wall Pilates

Wall Pilates frequently use specialized apparatus to enhance motions and provide additional support. The following are some key equipment commonly used in wall Pilates:

Wall

The wall is a crucial piece of equipment in Wall Pilates. It acts as a support and resistance tool, promoting stability and alignment during a wide range of activities.

Mat

A mat provides comfort and support, especially if your Wall Pilates practice involves floor exercises. It can also provide additional padding and define your workout area.

Contrary Bands:

Resistance bands can be used to add resistance to activities and intensify the workout. They are offered in varying intensities. They are versatile and effective at targeting various muscle groups.

Pilates sphere:

A stability ball, often known as a Pilates ball, generates a sense of instability, training core muscles and improving balance. Exercises against the wall are a frequent approach to assess stability.

Fit Ring Pilates (Magic Circle):

The Pilates ring is a flexible circle used to generate resistance for upper and lower body movements. It is used to increase difficulty and target certain muscle groups.

Yoga mats:

When necessary, yoga blocks can be utilized to modify postures and provide additional height or support. They are versatile and have numerous applications in Wall Pilates.

Grippy Footwear:

Wearing grip or non-slip socks may aid stability when working out against a wall. They provide traction and reduce the risk of slipping.

Weighted hand or dumbbells:

Depending on your fitness level, adding resistance to arm exercises using hand weights or dumbbells might make them more difficult for the upper body.

Ankle Straps:

The lower body can be strengthened and toned by adding resistance to leg movements with ankle weights wrapped around the ankles.

Pilates Handles:

Straps can be used to stretch and develop flexibility while practicing Wall Pilates. They can also help with specific workouts by supplying support as needed.

Anchor for the Pilates Wall:

A wall anchor may be required for some specific Wall Pilates exercises in order to securely tie resistance bands or other equipment to the wall.

Stopwatch or Timer:

Tracking the duration of your workout with a stopwatch or timer may be beneficial, especially if you're following a plan with predetermined intervals.

Before commencing a Wall Pilates workout, ensure that your equipment is properly set up and that you have everything you need. Adapt the resistance and intensity to your fitness level, and when completing exercises, always prioritize proper form and technique first.

Safety Considerations

Safety should always come first when performing Wall Pilates or any other type of activity. The following are some important safety factors to remember:

Speak to a Specialist:

Before beginning any new workout program, consult with a doctor or a professional fitness teacher to ensure that Wall Pilates is a good fit for you, particularly if you have any pre-existing health conditions.

The Right Warm-Up

Make sure you warm up adequately before starting any Wall Pilates session. By doing so, you reduce your risk of injury by preparing your muscles and joints for the workout.

Proper form:

When practicing exercises, focus on maintaining appropriate form. Proper alignment is required for successful activities and to avoid strain or damage.

Advance Gradually:

If you're new to Wall Pilates, start with beginner-friendly movements and progress to more demanding routines. This reduces the risk of overexertion and allows your body to adjust.

Take Note Of Your Body:

Observe how your body feels during and after each workout. Stop and assess if you have pain, which should not be confused with the regular soreness associated with exercise. Injuries may come from attempting to endure discomfort.

Use the appropriate tools:

Ensure that all of the equipment, such as stability balls and resistance bands, is in good working order and handled correctly. To ensure safety, follow the manufacturer's recommendations.

reliable anchors

If your Wall Pilates workout involves securing resistance bands or other gear to the wall, ensure that the wall anchors are firmly fastened. Before proceeding, ensure that the wall mount or attachment points are stable.

Make room.

To avoid falling or running into someone during an exercise, make sure the area around you is clear of barriers. Create a designated Pilates room to prevent potential risks.

Stay Hydrated:

Drink plenty of water when working out. Staying well hydrated improves overall health and minimizes fatigue.

Breath Consciousness:

Make sure you are breathing properly. Breathing promotes core engagement and increases oxygen flow to the muscles. When undertaking exercises, remember to breathe normally.

Adjust as necessary:

Be prepared to modify workouts based on any physical limitations or ailments you may have. Seek assistance from a fitness professional on appropriate changes.

Calm down:

Finish your Wall Pilates exercise with a complete cool-down to promote flexibility and allow your pulse rate to gradually return to normal.

Chapter 3

The Foundational Wall Pilates Exercises

Wall Pilates is a more playful version of regular Pilates. It takes core training routines to a new level by providing support in the shape of a wall or another hard surface. In contrast to traditional Pilates, which is based on gravity and body weight, Wall Pilates leverages the wall's strength to increase resistance.

Joseph Pilates, the bright man who developed the original Pilates method, came up with this groundbreaking concept. He would help his customers achieve proper alignment and form throughout their workouts by employing walls or other items. Today's instructors have taken those ideas and shaped Wall Pilates into what it is now.

The beauty of Wall Pilates stems from its incredible adaptability. Whether you're an experienced pro pushing the edge or a beginner laying the groundwork, there's something for everyone. With this simple regimen, you can say hello to defined arms, toned abs, and a booty that never fades.

Setting up the wall pillars

Pilates wall workouts require only a strong wall or a safe, smooth surface. Look for a space that is spacious enough for you to walk around and free of obstacles. You might also use a door with a dependable door stop as an anchor.

You'll need to warm up your body before beginning. Warming up can help prepare your muscles, boost blood flow, and prevent injuries. Thus, spend five to ten minutes doing a modest dynamic warm-up that includes cardio and light stretches.

When you're ready, let's get started on some excellent Wall Pilates exercises. Feel the motions, accept the wall's support, and maintain good posture. Remember to work your core like a boss during each workout. Before attempting more difficult techniques, take your time establishing the proper form and stance.

Essential Workouts for Wall Pilates

SAMPLE ROLL-DOWN WALL

This is a must-do exercise for stretching your spine and strengthening your core.

Place your feet six to ten inches apart, with your back to the wall. Keep your arms straight, shoulders down, and chest wide while squeezing your abs.

Inhale deeply, nod your head, and slowly roll down, feeling the separation of each vertebra. Your arms remain aligned with your ears. Continue until your hips are stationary against the wall.

Breathe in and feel the stretch. Now, exhale and roll back up, resting each vertebra against the wall with your lower abs.

Pay attention to the time when your upper torso rolls up between your shoulders. And just like that, shoulders lowered and abs engaged, returning to the starting posture.

WALL SKIN

Place your forearms on the wall and form a plank position, keeping your body straight from head to heels.

Maintain that posture by contracting your shoulders, glutes, and abs.

Would you like to heighten it? Stabilize your hips and perform leg lifts or shoulder taps.

Wall plank variations engage your shoulders and stabilizer muscles while strengthening and conditioning your core.

FRONT BRIDGE

This workout focuses on improving core stability and shaping the glutes and low back.

Lie on your back with your feet pressed against the wall and your knees comfortably bent at a 90-degree angle.

Elevate your hips off the floor, tuck your arms by your sides, and press your feet against the wall.

Maintain an erect stance from shoulder to knee. Squeeze your glutes and lower back while holding the bridge for a short time, then slowly lower your hips back down.

These intense Wall Pilates workouts are ideal for building a strong core and increasing your sexy body awareness. After you've mastered the foundations, you can go on to more challenging Wall Pilates routines.

PURPOSE OF WALL PILATES

Perhaps you're wondering whether wall Pilates is beneficial. We'll tell you: the answer is absolutely yes! These are some incredible benefits of this enticing activity.

Essential Structure and Stability

The purpose of this workout is to build amazing core strength. Your lower back, obliques, and deep abdominal muscles can all help to develop and stabilize your core. You'll be unstoppable in other pursuits, but you'll also have perfect posture and no lower back problems.

OPTIMIZED VERSATILITY

Wall Pilates routines provide a blend of static and dynamic stretches, increasing your flexibility to unimaginable levels. As you advance through these exercises, your range of motion will gradually increase, allowing you to move freely throughout your everyday activities.

Enhanced posture

Postural imbalances can be addressed, and an appealing upright posture can be acquired by focusing on alignment and body awareness. Reducing persistent back and neck pain entails strengthening the muscles that keep you in alignment.

Low-impact workouts

Wall Pilates is suitable for people of all ages and fitness levels due to its gentleness on the joints. This workout is ideal for individuals who wish to exercise without stress or are recovering from an illness.

IMPROVE YOUR FITNESS WITH WALL PILATES.

Wall Pilates offers a comprehensive and revolutionary approach to physical training. It has the potential to alter people's lives at any fitness level. To get the wonderful benefits of this unconventional exercise, accept the focused motions, set achievable goals, and practice consistently.

The Gentle Warm-Up Movements

It's critical to warm up carefully before beginning any workout, including Wall Pilates. The following are some simple warm-up exercises to prepare your body for a Wall Pilates lesson.
Chin and Neck Rolls:
To release tension, slowly swivel your head side to side, then gently roll your neck clockwise and counterclockwise.

Backwards Rolls:

Circularly move your shoulders back and forth. This helps relieve stress in the upper back and shoulder joints.

Arm Rotation:

Make little circles in both directions while extending your arms to the sides. As you warm up your shoulder muscles, gradually widen the circles.

Torso rotations:

Spread your feet hip-width apart and twist your torso in a smooth circular motion. Maintain control of your movements by staying within a comfortable range.

Side Curves:

While standing or sitting, raise one arm and slowly bend your torso to the opposite side. Repetition on the opposing side will extend your sides.

Circular hips:

Place your feet hip-width apart and spin your hips clockwise and counterclockwise while standing. This promotes hip joint warmth.

Leg raises:

Raise your knees to your chest while standing, as if marching. This improves circulation and contracts the muscles in your legs.

Wrist Rolls:

Raise one foot off the ground while sitting or standing. Turn your ankle to the side and back. Change to the opposite foot. This helps to warm up your lower legs and ankles.

Grasping circles:

Stretch your arms out in front of you, doing circular movements with your wrists. This is especially useful for Wall Pilates techniques that require your hands to be involved.

Cat-Cow Exercise:

If you're on the ground, go to your hands and knees. Take a deep breath, lift your head, and arch your back (Cow position). Exhale, arch your back, and raise your chin to your chest (cat position). Repeat.

March in Position:

Gently march in place while raising your knees. This warms the lower body and gradually boosts the heart rate.

Deep inhalation:

Breathe deeply through your diaphragm to increase the flow of oxygen to your muscles. Exhale slowly through your lips after inhaling deeply through your nose and squeezing your diaphragm.

Take your time with these warm-up exercises so that your body can adjust to action after rest. An appropriate warm-up increases flexibility, reduces the risk of injury, and prepares your body and mind for the following Wall Pilates movements.

Core-Strengthening Techniques

One of the primary aims of Pilates, particularly Wall Pilates, is core strength. You can incorporate the following core-strengthening exercises into your routine:
Pelvic Heave:
Lie on your back, feet hip-width apart, knees bent. To begin, take a breath, exhale, and engage your abdominal muscles to lift your pelvis. Take some time to hold, then let go. Repeat.

Leg lifts:

Extend your legs while lying on your back. Raise one leg toward the ceiling while keeping the other on the ground. The lifted leg should be lowered without touching the floor. Alternate your legs deliberately.

Crunches on bikes:

Put your hands behind your head and lie on your back. Raising your legs off the floor, bend one knee toward your chest and twist your torso such that the opposite elbow is directed toward that knee. Swap sides when pedaling.

Changes in planks

Maintain a typical plank posture, with your arms straight. Maintain a straight posture and activate your core. Side planks are another alternative for more indirect activity.

Taking a Ball-like Roll:

Take a seat on the mat, knees tucked into your chest, and balance on your sit bones. Roll backward while holding your ankles, then step back to restore your balance. This puts your central control system at danger.

One hundred:

Stretch your arms forwards, lift your legs off the ground, and lie on your back. As you raise and drop your arms, breathe in for five counts, then out for five counts. This strenuous exercise works the core and boosts stamina.

The Swan Dive

Lying face down, arms extended front. Taking a deep inhale, lift your arms, legs, and torso off the floor all at once. To protect your neck, keep your head down. Exhale as you drop again.

Side Leg Extensions:

While lying on your side, use your forearm to support your upper body. Raise your upper leg, then lower it down. This targets the oblique and outer hip muscles.

Russian Twist in the Seat:

Take a seat on the mat, knees bowed and feet flat. Lean back slightly while maintaining a straight back. Twist your torso to one side, then the other, keeping your hands together.

The Saw

Stretch your legs out to be slightly wider than hip-width apart while sitting, then stretch your arms to the sides. Twist your torso and reach your opposing hand to the outside of the opposing foot.

Double Leg Extensions:

Raise your head and shoulders off the mat while resting on your back with your knees against your chest. Your arms and legs should be extended straight out, then brought back in towards your chest.

Scissors Practice:

Stretch both legs toward the ceiling while resting on your back. Then, lower one leg to the floor while keeping the other high. In a scissor-like motion, switch legs.

Leg and Arm Exercises for Beginners

You can incorporate Wall Pilates and other beginner-friendly arm and leg movements into your Pilates routine by performing the following:
Leg Warm-Up: Wall Sit.

Stand with your back against the wall and squat down with your knees bent 90 degrees. Hold for as long as you feel comfortable contracting your glutes and thighs.

Legs pressed toward the wall

Lie on your back, legs bent and feet braced on the wall. Legs straightened by pressing your feet against the wall should be bent back to their original posture.

Marching to the ready:

Assume a tall stance by raising your legs to your chest while marching. This is a low-impact exercise that activates your hip flexors and raises leg temperature.

Side Leg Extensions:

Assume a side-prone position and rest your head on your lower arm. Reach up toward the ceiling with the upper leg, then lower it. This works on the thighs and outer hips.

Slides with heels:

Bend your knees and lie back. To straighten the leg, slide one heel along the mat and then bend it back to its original position. Swap the legs.

Arm Workout:

Bench Press Ups:

Position yourself such that your hands are shoulder height away from the wall. Bend your elbows, lower your chest on the wall, and then push back up to the beginning position.

Arm Rotation:

Raise your arms shoulder-high to the sides. With your arms, gradually extend the small circles you've created. Rotate the circles in the other way.

Resistance Band Bicep Curls:

Sit or stand on the resistance band, grasping one end with each hand. Curling your hands toward your shoulders will engage your biceps. Reposition them lower.

Tricep dips:

Sit on the chair's edge, grasping the front edge with your hands. Lower your body by bending your elbows and sliding your hips off the chair. Pushing up returns you to the starting position.

Arm lifts:

Hold your arms at your sides and stand. Raise both arms to shoulder height and then lower them back down. Repeat this to develop your shoulder muscles.

Press your shoulders on the wall.

Face the wall, holding your arms at shoulder height. Straighten your arms and press your palms against the wall.

Grasping circles:

Stretch your arms out in front of you, doing circular movements with your wrists. This promotes forearm and wrist warmth.

Hand Plank:

Begin in a plank position with your forearms. Maintain a straight posture and use your arms and core to support your body.

During these exercises, focus on proper form, control, and breathing. Increase the number of reps gradually as your strength improves. If you have any worries or medical conditions, you should consult a fitness expert or healthcare provider before starting a new workout plan.

Chapter 4

Building Strength and Flexibility

Building both strength and flexibility is beneficial to overall fitness and well-being. Here's a well-rounded set of beginner-friendly exercises to help you develop both strength and flexibility:

Exercises to Build Strength:

Weightlifting Squats:

Form a squat by placing your feet hip-width apart, raising your chest, and bending your knees so they are over your toes. Put pressure on your heels to return to your starting position.

Step-Ups:

Begin in a plank position, bending your elbows to lower your body and then pushing yourself back up. If necessary, perform wall push-ups.

Pleuces:

Begin with one foot front and squat down until your knees are 90 degrees bent. Push yourself back up to the starting position, then repeat with the second leg.

Board:

Maintain a plank position, with your torso aligned from head to heels. Hold as long as possible while engaging your core.

Exercise for Bridge:

Assume a prone position, bend your knees, raise your hips to the ceiling, and clench your glutes at the top. Position your hips lower.

Barbell rows:

Squeeze your shoulder blades together while holding a dumbbell in each hand, hunching down at the hips and rowing the weights to your chest.

Exercises for flexibility:

Folding forward:

Place your feet hip-width apart and extend your hips to the ground. Stretch your spine and relieve tension in your head and neck.

Hip flexor extension:

Drop to one knee and gently press your hips forward, keeping your other foot in front of you. Your hips should feel stretched in front of you.

Leaning forward in the seat:

Sit with your legs extended, flex your hips, and reach for your toes. Maintain a straight back and avoid bending your spine.

Stretch For Chest Openers:

Raise your arms straight, clasp them behind your back, and open your chest slightly. Take deep breaths while holding the stretch.

Infant Pose:

Beggin on your hands and knees, then extend your arms forward while sitting back on your heels. This will cause your shoulders and back muscles to flex.

Cat-Cow Exercise:

While on your hands and knees, lift your head and tailbone (cow) by arching your back and lowering your belly. Repeat this fluid movement.

Butterfly Extension:

Sit with your legs bent outward and your soles together. Hold your feet and move your knees slightly toward the floor to stretch your inner thighs.

Tricep Extension:

Gently press your second hand against your bent elbow after stretching one hand down your back between your shoulder blades. To extend both triceps, swap arms.

Progressive Exercises for Muscle Endurance

Increasing the length or intensity of workouts gradually over time is essential for improving muscle endurance. To improve overall muscle endurance, attempt this progressive set of workouts that target multiple muscle groups:

Body Below:

Weightlifting Squats:

Start with two sets of 15-20 squats. As you become more comfortable, gradually increase the amount of repetitions.

Pleuces:

Begin with two sets of 10 lunges per leg. As you progress, increase the number of lunges you do or attempt new ones, such as walking lunges.

Next steps:

Use a stable step or platform. Start by doing 12 step-ups in each leg twice. As your strength improves, increase the number of sets or step height.

Wall pose:

As your endurance improves, steadily increase the duration of your 30-second wall sit.

Upper Region:

Step-Ups:

Start with two sets of ten push-ups. Increase the number of push-ups gradually or progress to harder variations.

Barbell rows:

Begin each arm with two sets of twelve rows. As your strength improves, increase the amount of repetitions or utilize heavier weight.

Tricep dips:

Start with two sets of twelve tricep dips. Make sure you maintain appropriate form. Make progress by increasing the difficulty or amount of repeats.

Crabbe curls:

Begin with two sets of 15 light dumbbell bicep curls. As your endurance improves, progressively increase the weight or number of reps.

Main:

Board:

Begin with two sets of 30-60 seconds. Gradually extend the duration. Remember to maintain your body straight from head to heels.

Russian parodies:

Begin with 20 twists, two sets of 10 on each side. As your core strength improves, increase the weight or repetitions.

Leg lifts:

Start with two sets of twelve leg lifts. For an added difficulty, increase the number of sets or slow down the movement.

Crunches on bikes:

Begin with 15 bike crunches, separated into two sets. Try adding extra repetitions or variations, such as double leg bicycles.

Heart-related endurance:

Jacks with Jumps:

Begin with two sets of 30-60 seconds. Gradually increase the duration to improve cardiovascular endurance.

Lifted knees:

Begin with two 30 second sets. As you progress, raise your knees further to increase the time or intensity of the exercise.

Push-ups:

Do two sets of five burpees to begin. To raise the intensity, perform a push-up or increase the amount of reps.

Jog or Run:

Begin with 10 to 15 minutes, then gradually increase the duration as your cardiovascular endurance improves.

Stretching Into Wall Pilates

Stretching is an excellent technique to improve your range of motion, flexibility, and the effectiveness of your Wall Pilates practice. You can incorporate the following stretches into your Wall Pilates session:
Wall Chest Extension:
Hold your hands at shoulder height and face the wall. Feel the stretch in your shoulders and chest as you bend forward and place your palms on the wall.

Hip Flexor Wall Stretch:

Turn to face the wall and place your hands there. Retrace one step, keeping your heel on the ground. Bend your front knee to feel a stretch in the hip flexor of the extended leg.

Flex your wall hamstrings.

Take a seat near the wall, one leg pulled up against it. Feel the stretch at the back of your extended leg as you lean forward and reach for your toes.

Calf Extension:

Place your hands against the wall as you face it. Retrace one foot while maintaining a straight gait. Feel your calf stretch as you plant your heel into the ground.

Shoulder-to-wall stretch:

As you stand, raise one arm shoulder-high against the wall. Turn your body away from the wall to gently stretch your shoulders and chest.

Twist of Wall Spine:

Sit on the ground with your side against the wall. Feel the strain in your obliques and spine as you rotate your torso while holding one hand against the wall.

Cat-Cow Wall Stretch:

Position yourself such that your hands are shoulder height away from the wall. Drop your tummy to arch your back (cow), then tuck your chin in and round your back (cat).

Stretch your wall quadriceps.

Take a stand facing the wall, using it for support. Bend one knee and move your heel toward your glutes, then grip your foot with your palm to stretch your quadriceps.

Stretching for Wall Lateral Flexion:

While standing sideways against the wall, place your hand at shoulder height. Raise your opposite arm above your head to perform a lateral stretch along your side.

The Wall Child Pose

Reach your arms forward along the wall, kneeling with your back to it and sitting on your heels. This stretches your arms and lengthens your spine.

Adapting Movements to Your Fitness Level

To be both safe and effective, an exercise's motions must be tailored to your present fitness level. These are common concepts for changing movements in a Wall Pilates routine, regardless of ability level:

For novices:

Reduced Motion Range:

When exercising, begin with a lesser range of motion and progressively develop your strength and flexibility. This is especially important for movements of the shoulders, hips, and back.

Supportive adjustments:

Use accessories or modifications to help. For example, use a chair or a stability ball to assist you keep balanced while executing certain exercises.

Repetition Reduction:

Begin with fewer repetitions or less time spent in each pose. As you become more comfortable with the moves, progressively increase the duration and intensity.

Easier exercises:

Opt for easier exercise variations. Choose easy squats, for example, before progressing to more challenging leg workouts against a wall.

Put Form First:

Prioritize alignment and proper form over intensity. This is critical for establishing a stable foundation and preventing accidents.

For Levels In Between:

Extend your range of motion during exercises to help your muscles work harder. This can include longer arm exercises against the wall, deeper squats, and larger leg lifts.

Progressive Resistance: To improve exercises, progressively increase resistance by using light hand weights or resistance bands.

Increased repetitions or sets: Increase the number of repetitions or sets. This improves your muscles' stamina and endurance.

Combination and Variation:

Try different workout modifications and combining routines to make the exercises more difficult. For an added difficulty, consider twisting leg lifts, for example.

Balance Exercises: Additional balancing exercises, such as one-legged poses against the wall, can help increase stability and core activation.

For Levels Upward:

The full range of motion

When completing exercises, aim to employ your whole range of motion to optimize muscle contraction and stretch. This is especially crucial for advanced Pilates routines done against a wall.

Increased resistance: To make strength training more difficult, employ thicker resistance bands or heavier weights.

Advanced variations: Incorporating twists, pulses, or combining motions into your Pilates exercises can provide a more dynamic and challenging workout.

High Repetition Sets: High repetition sets will help you build muscle endurance. This may mean performing a series of exercises with little to no rest in between sets.

Flow and fluidity: Maintain a smooth transition between exercises, focusing on the control and correctness of each action. This promotes enhanced muscular engagement and increases coordination.

Pay attention to your body and don't push yourself beyond your comfort zone, regardless of your fitness level. If an exercise appears too challenging, return to a more basic form or make changes as needed. If the workout appears to be too easy, progress to a more tougher version. Routinely reevaluating and changing your regimen can ensure that you continue to develop and avoid plateaus on your fitness path. If you have any health issues or concerns, consult with a fitness specialist.

Chapter 5

Create Your Wall Pilates Routine

By creating a personalized Wall Pilates program, you can tailor your workout to your fitness level, preferences, and goals. Here's a step-by-step tutorial to help you construct your Wall Pilates routine:

1. Set precise goals.

Decide on your fitness goals, such as core stability, strength, flexibility, or overall health. Setting specific goals will help you plan your time.

2. Exercise:

Begin your practice with a short warm-up to prepare your muscles and joints for the workouts. Incorporate dynamic workouts like arm circles, leg swings, and neck tilts.

3. Basic Workouts:

Include a range of wall-based core strengthening activities. This may include exercises such as wall sits, leg raises, and bicycle crunches. Try to blend exercises that target different sections of your core in a balanced manner.

4. Upper Body Workouts

Incorporate upper-body exercises such as dumbbell rows against the wall, wall push-ups, and wall shoulder stretches. Incorporate exercises that target the arms, back, shoulders, and chest.

5. Abdominal Exercise:

Include lower-body exercises like step-ups, wall squats, and wall hip flexor stretches. Make sure your strategy is comprehensive, focusing on various leg and gluteal muscle groups.

6. Stretching for Flexibility:

A portion of your workout should be dedicated to wall stretching. Workouts like the wall quadriceps stretch, wall hamstring stretch, and wall chest stretch can help you improve your range of motion and flexibility.

7. Equilibrium Activities:

Include balancing exercises to improve your stability. To strengthen your core and lower body, try one-legged poses against a wall or other balancing activities.

8. Exercises with Pilates ball and resistance bands:

If you have Pilates props available, consider including workouts with a Pilates ball or resistance bands. This may intensify some movements and provide diversity.

9. Inhaling and Becoming Aware

Maintain focus on your breathing throughout the workout. Pilates pushes you to breathe carefully while performing each action. This promotes relaxation while also boosting the exercise's efficacy.

10. De-stress.

- Finish your workout with a cool-down to promote flexibility and help your heart rate gradually return to normal. Make sure to include wall stretches for all major muscle groups.

11. Development and Adjustment:

Evaluate your progress and fitness level on a regular basis. Exercises can be made more challenging by introducing new variations, increasing repetitions, or modifying intensity as needed.

A example routine for wall Pilates:

Assemble:

Arm circles, leg swings, and neck tilts (5 min.)

Core workouts:

Wall Sit for two 30-second sets.

Leg Lifts: 2 sets (12 total)

Bike Crunches (15 sets total).

Upper body workouts:

Ten wall pushups in two sets.

Row with dumbbells against the wall, two sets of twelve per arm.

Wall shoulder exercise: One 30-second set.

Lower body workouts:

Wall climbs (15 sets total)

Wall Hip Flexor Stretch: 30 seconds per leg, separated into one set.

Step-ups: two sets (12 reps for each leg).

Stretching and Flexibility:

Stretch the wall chest once for thirty seconds.

Wall Hamstring Exercise: One 30-second set.

Stretching the wall quadriceps: one set of thirty seconds each leg.

Balance Activities:

Pose with one leg against the wall for two sets (20 seconds for each leg).

Exercises with a Pilates ball and resistance bands:

Exercise Ball Squeezes (2 sets of 15)

Pull-Aparts with Resistance Bands (two sets of twelve)

Inhaling and Becoming Aware

Pilates breathing emphasizes controlled and rhythmic breathing.

Calm down:

Bending forward while seated against a wall for one set of thirty seconds.

Child's Pose: One 30-second set with your forehead against the wall.

Always remember to tailor the program to your own demands and progress gradually as your fitness level improves. If you are new to the activity or have any health concerns, consult with a fitness expert or healthcare provider before starting a new training plan.

How To Design a Personalized Workout Plan

Creating a personalized training plan for wall Pilates requires taking into account your fitness goals, current fitness level, any physical constraints, and personal preferences. Here's a step-by-step approach to help you design a personalized plan:

Determine Your Fitness Goals: Decide what you want to accomplish with your wall Pilates workouts. Do you want to enhance core strength, flexibility, posture, or general fitness? Your goals will influence how your training regimen is structured.

Evaluate your fitness level. Determine your current level of fitness, including strength, flexibility, and endurance. This examination will help you select appropriate exercises and progressions.

Consult with a professional. If you are new to Pilates or have any health concerns, you should speak with a trained Pilates instructor or fitness professional. They may offer advice suited to your individual needs and goals, assuring safety and efficacy.

Select Wall Pilates Exercises: Wall Pilates combines traditional Pilates exercises with the support of a wall. Choose a variety of exercises that work different muscle groups and movement patterns. Wall squats, leg lifts, bridges, and wall angels are some of the most common Pilates exercises.

Plan your workout structure: Create a systematic workout regimen that includes a warm-up, primary exercise, and cool-down. Strive for a balance of strength, flexibility, and stability exercises. Consider combining dynamic movements with static holds.

Set Reps and Sets: Determine the number of repetitions and sets for each exercise based on your fitness level and objectives. Beginners can start with 2-3 sets of 8-12 repetitions each exercise, while more advanced athletes can aim for greater repetitions or more sets.

Progression and Variation: As you become more familiar with the exercises, progressively increase their intensity, duration, or complexity to keep your body challenged and progressing. You can also add modifications or advanced versions of exercises to keep your training interesting.

Include Rest Days: Allow for enough rest and recovery time between workouts to avoid overtraining and enhance muscle recovery. Listen to your body and alter the frequency of your workouts accordingly.

Listen to your body. Pay attention to how your body reacts to the workouts. If you suffer any pain or discomfort, alter the workout or consult with a specialist. It is critical to prioritize safety and avoid pushing oneself too hard.

Monitor Your Progress: Keep note of your exercise, noting any increases in strength, flexibility, or endurance over time. To continue making progress toward your goals, adjust your training schedule accordingly.

Stay Consistent: Consistency is essential for seeing benefits with any fitness routine. Aim to add wall Pilates into your daily routine and make it a habit for long-term results.

Combining Exercises for Full-Body Engagement

Combining exercises that target different muscle groups is essential for creating a workout that works your entire body. This is a total-body fitness program that combines cardiovascular, strength, and flexibility training.

1. Warm-up with two one-minute bouts of jumping jacks.

Arm circles: two 30-second sets each direction

Two one-minute sets for high knees.

2. Cardiovascular Activity: twenty minutes of brisk walking or running.

Take breaks (30 seconds of vigorous activity, followed by 30 seconds of moderate activity).

3. Exercise for Strength:

Three sets of fifteen squats.

Push-ups: three 12 rep sets.

Three sets of twelve lunges per leg.

Dumbbell bent-over rows, three sets of twelve

4. Core Workouts: 3 sets of 30 seconds of plank

Three sets of twenty Russian twists (10 on each side)

3 sets of 15 bicycle crunches per side.

5. Balance and flexibility: Forward fold: Two sets of 30 seconds.

Warrior II position: two 30-second sets each.

Tree Pose: 30-second sets for each leg.

6. Full-body Exercise: Three sets of 10 burpees.

7. Child pose: two sets of thirty seconds.

Stretch your chest against the wall for two sets of 30 seconds.

Cat-cow stretches: two one-minute sets.

Remarks:

When practicing strength training activities, make sure to use controlled movements and proper technique.

Match the intensity to your level of fitness. Make any required adjustments to the number of sets or repetitions.

If required, add rest intervals between sets and exercises.

Stay hydrated throughout your workout.

This program incorporates a variety of exercises to target different muscle groups, promote flexibility, and improve cardiovascular fitness. Always pay attention to your body, and if you have any pre-existing medical concerns, consult with a healthcare professional or fitness specialist before starting a new workout routine.

My Secret for Consistency and Progress Tracking

Tracking progress and keeping consistency are two critical components of any successful fitness regimen. The following suggestions will help you maintain consistency and easily track your progress:

Continuity:

Set sensible goals:

Set realistic long-term and short-term goals. Setting and completing realistic goals will keep you motivated and on track.

Establish a timetable:

Plan your workouts ahead of time and include them into your weekly schedule. Approach exercise as a required component of your routine, no different than any other commitment.

Locate Pleasurable Activities

Choose physical activities and workouts you enjoy. You're more likely to stick to a fitness routine if you enjoy it.

Blend it Up:

Change up your workouts to avoid boredom. Include a range of workouts, such as aerobics, strength training, flexibility, and balance exercises.

To improve accountability, consider working out with a friend or joining a fitness class. Having someone anticipate your needs can boost your dedication.

Gradual Progression: After establishing a manageable baseline, progressively increase the duration or intensity of your workouts. This reduces the risk of harm and helps to prevent burnout.

Progress Monitoring

Maintain a workout log:

Keep track of all the exercises, sets, repetitions, and mental notes you take during your workout. This journal can be a great tool for tracking your progress over time.

Measure it out:

Measure physical changes in your body, such as waist, hip, and body fat percentage, in addition to your weight. These measures may, on occasion, better reflect your progress.

Frequent evaluations: Evaluate your strength, flexibility, and cardiovascular health on a regular basis. Use benchmarks to track progress and identify areas that require additional work.

Fitness apps can help you schedule routines, set goals, and track your progress. Numerous apps include features for tracking food, keeping track of workouts, and logging exercises.

Progress Photos: Take before and after photos of your physique to see the changes. Seeing the improvement in this way may be inspirational, even if it is not obvious on a scale.

Honor Significant Occasions:

Congratulate yourself on your achievements, whether it's completing a challenging workout, reducing weight, or performing better. Positive reinforcement motivates people.

Take note of your body's sensations and functioning. Positive progress is evidenced by improved attitude, sleep, and vitality.

Frequent visits:

Schedule regular self-evaluations to track your progress toward fitness. Evaluate your goals, adjust your strategy as necessary, and acknowledge your progress as it occurs.

Remember that there will be ups and downs, and growth is not always linear. Patience, persistence, and a positive attitude are key components of a successful fitness journey. Celebrate your progress towards a better, more active lifestyle, and make any required changes to your strategy.

Chapter 6

The Advanced wall Pilate Exercises

Wall Push up Work

Wall push-ups primarily target the triceps, shoulders, and chest. Because they put less strain on the upper body than normal floor push-ups, they're an excellent workout for beginners or those aiming to develop their upper body.

Leaning against the wall and pushing your body away activates the pectoralis major (chest muscle), anterior deltoids (front shoulder muscles), and triceps brachii (back of the arm muscles). The serratus anterior (the muscles around the ribs) as well as the core muscles are employed to stabilize the body during movement.

Wall push-ups are an excellent activity to incorporate into your workout routine if you want to improve your upper body strength, muscle endurance, and overall functional fitness. As you gain strength, you can go to more challenging push-up variations such as floor push-ups or incline push-ups.
Engaging Muscles: Wall push-ups are primarily designed to work upper-body muscles such as the triceps, shoulders, and chest. The pectoralis major, the largest muscle in the chest, is heavily employed when pushing against the wall. Furthermore, the muscles at the front of the shoulder, known as the anterior deltoids, and the back of the arm, known as the triceps brachii, are essential for performing the exercise.

One of the key advantages of wall push-ups is that they are easy to do and suitable for beginners. Wall push-ups are less taxing on the upper body than typical floor push-ups, making them a more manageable place to begin for persons new to strength training or those who struggle with floor exercises. Because less body weight must be raised in the inclined position against the wall, the exercise is easier to accomplish with proper technique.

Stabilization and Core Engagement: While wall push-ups primarily train the upper body muscles, they also work the serratus anterior, or muscles surrounding the rib cage, as well as the core muscles to help stabilize the body during the activity. Maintaining a straight line from the head to the heels and avoiding excessive arching or lowering of the back will effectively engage the core muscles and improve overall stability.

Progression and Variation: As people become stronger and more proficient at wall push-ups, they can add new push-up variations or adjust the angle at which their body is positioned in respect to the wall to gradually increase the difficulty. To engage more muscles and enhance strength and stability, try inclining the body at a steeper angle or performing push-ups on an unstable surface (such as a stability ball).

Benefits of Functional Fitness: Wall push-ups have practical applications in everyday tasks and functional motions, as well as helping to increase upper-body strength and muscle endurance. Strong arms, shoulders, and chest muscles are required for tasks such as moving objects, lifting, and carrying groceries, as well as maintaining excellent posture and upper body alignment during a variety of activities.

Wall push-ups are an excellent complement to any workout routine, particularly for novices or those seeking a low-impact technique to build their upper body. They are an effective workout for improving upper-body strength, muscle tone, and general functional fitness.

Single Leg Wall Bridge

The single-leg wall bridge is a more difficult variation on the standard wall bridge exercise that develops the core, hamstrings, and glutes while improving stability and balance. Here's how to do it:

Position your feet hip-width apart and flat against the wall while lying on your back. For stability, keep your arms by your sides.

Lift Hips: To lift your hips off the ground and form a straight line from your shoulders to your knees, engage your core and apply pressure to your heels.

Single Leg Lift: After you've positioned yourself in the bridge pose, elevate one leg off the ground and straight ahead of you. Keep your toes pointed upward and your lifted leg aligned with your hips.

Hold and Lower: Keep your hips level and steady while keeping the single-leg bridge stance for a short time. Finally, return your lifted leg to the wall.

Repeat with the Other Leg: Lift the other leg off the wall while maintaining the bridge position with the same motion.

Whole Repetitions: Lift each leg alternately for the desired number of reps or duration, ensuring flawless form at all times.

This workout improves unilateral strength, balance, and stability while also challenging the glutes, hamstrings, and core muscles. As your strength and stability improve, gradually increase the amount of repetitions you do on each leg from the start.

Hamstring and gluteal muscle activation: The main muscles employed during the single-leg wall bridge exercise are the gluteus maximus, the largest muscle in the buttocks, and the hamstrings, which are located at the back of the thigh. Raising one leg off the wall while maintaining the bridge position increases the tension on the hip stabilizing muscles and works your hamstrings and glutes harder than a conventional wall bridge.

Core Stability and Engagement: To maintain proper alignment and avoid excessive arching or sagging of the lower back, the single-leg variant of the wall bridge, like the classic version, requires strong core stability and engagement. The deep core muscles, including the obliques and transverse abdominis, help to build a strong and sturdy foundation. These muscles serve to support the pelvis and spine.

Unilateral Strength and Balance: To treat muscle imbalances between the left and right sides, execute exercises that focus on one side of the body at a time, such as the single-leg wall bridge. Lifting one leg off the wall increases the tension on the standing leg's stabilizing muscles, which improves general balance and proprioception (awareness of body position in space).

Walking, running, and jumping are common activities and sports that need unilateral lower body strength and stability. The single-leg wall bridge mimics these movements and barriers. Strengthening the muscles involved in functional duties can help you perform better and reduce your risk of injury.

Progression and Variation: As you gain strength and competence in the single-leg wall bridge, you may push yourself harder by including more variants into the exercise. For example, you can execute the exercise on an unstable surface, such as a stability ball or foam roller, to test your stability and balance, or you can hold a weight or resistance band across your hips for added resistance.

Safety and Correct Form: To reduce the risk of injury and maximize efficacy, maintain proper form throughout the workout. Avoid twisting or tilting your pelvis; instead, focus on keeping level and firm hips. Furthermore, to support your lower back and keep your spine in a neutral position, activate your core muscles throughout the movement.

Use the single-leg wall bridge as part of your regular strength training routine to develop your core, hamstrings, and glutes. It also helps you gain balance, stability, and functional strength. As you develop and become more comfortable with the exercise, gradually increase the amount of repetitions you perform on each leg from the start.

Wall Plank

The wall plank, a take on the traditional plank exercise, uses the shoulders, arms, and legs for stability in addition to working the core muscles including the lower back, obliques, and abdominals. You go about it like this:

Put your hands on the wall, little wider than shoulder-width apart, with your back to the wall. Adjust your feet such that your body forms a straight line from your head to your heels and your arms are out in front of you.

Check that your wrists are precisely beneath your shoulders and that your feet are hip-width apart. Utilizing your core muscles to prevent your lower back from slumping, maintain your neck in line with your spine and your head down toward the floor.

Hold: Keep your body in a straight line and your core muscles engaged by staying in the plank position as long as you'd like. Breathe deeply and regularly all through the exercise, not holding your breath.

Alternatives: If you find the wall plank too challenging, you can ease the difficulty by putting your hands on a solid bench or countertop or by bringing your feet closer to the wall to reduce the angle of your torso.

Step your feet farther away from the wall to increase the angle at which your body is positioned as your strength grows, or lift one leg off the wall to generate more instability and further work your stabilizing muscles.

The wall plank is a versatile exercise that can be included into your regimen to strengthen your core, boost your balance and stability, and raise your level of general functional fitness. Hold the plank briefly at first, then gradually increase the time as your endurance and strength grow.

Wall Pick

Actually, "Wall Pick" is a sophisticated Pilates exercise that uses the knees and shoulders to give stability in addition to working the obliques and abdominals specifically. You go about it like this:

Laying on your back, with your legs out in front of you and your arms at your sides, is the initial setup. Settle down close to a wall, your legs stretched upward toward the ceiling and your feet flat on the wall. Pull in your core muscles to maintain stability in your spine.

Breathe in to warm up, then exhale as you straighten and lift your legs off the wall. You should be rising with your feet pointing up at the ceiling.

Pelvic Lift: Keeping your hips off the mat and exhaling, curl your tailbone toward your knees and tighten your lower abdominals. Press your arms down into the mat firmly for further stability.

Wall Pick: As you raise your hips as high as you can without sacrificing control, feel your core muscles contract for a brief period of time.

Lowering: Inhale to slowly lower your hips to the mat and return to the starting position.

Repeat: Keeping careful attention to your precise and controlled movements, complete the activity as many times as you choose.

The Wall Pick strains the abdominal and pelvic muscles by making them lift the legs and hips off the mat against gravity's resistance. It also builds the muscles in the shoulders and upper back and promotes hamstring flexibility.

You have to keep good form and alignment throughout this advanced Pilates exercise to prevent strain or injury. As your control and strength increase, up the amount of repetitions. Give a few a start. If you are new to Pilates or have any underlying health issues, you should consult with a qualified instructor before starting advanced exercises like the Wall Pick.

Wall Abdominal Curl

A challenging Pilates exercise, the "Wall Abdominal Curl" stimulates the abdominal muscles, especially the rectus abdominis, or "six-pack" muscles, as well as the hip flexors and pelvic floor muscles. You go about it like this:

Setup: Sit with your back against a wall, feet level and hip-width apart. Your lower back should stay in contact with the wall the whole workout.

To use your core muscles, keep your pelvis neutral and move your navel toward your spine.

Arm Position: Holding your palms together, extend your arms parallel to the ground straight out in front of you. Use of this arm position maintains balance and stability throughout the activity.

As you progressively bend your upper body forward, curling your spine away from the wall one vertebra at a time, take a breath to warm up. Pull your ribs in toward your pelvis; do not arch your lower back.

Reach and Hold: Keep curling forward until your abdominal muscles clench firmly. When you reach your hands toward your feet, try not to strain or tug at your neck.

Breath out, then slowly and deliberately roll back down, articulating your spine one vertebrae at a time against the wall. All through the workout, keep your core engaged.

Repeat: Curl the desired amount of times, being sure to move deliberately and under control.

The Wall Abdominal Curl examines the abdominal muscles and allows a closer look at spinal articulation and core activation because of the wall's support. Maintaining proper form the entire time will help to avoid straining your neck or lower back.

Just as with any workout, start with a few reps and increase them as your control and strength increase. If you are new to Pilates or have any underlying health issues, it is best to speak with a qualified instructor to ensure perfect technique and make any required adjustments.

Chapter 7

5 Simple Practical EXERCISES

ONE-SIDED WALL SLIDING

With a one-sided wall sliding mechanism, you may cleverly slide a panel or door parallel to one wall. In modern constructions, it's a standard arrangement for partitioning living rooms or hiding unutilized spaces.

Resources and Tools You Will Need

directing wheel
Murals for the walls
Rolling terrain
Systems of fastening
Fasteners in general
Tape for measuring drilling levels
Screwdriver Setup Measure the wall's length and width to be sure the panel or door fits correctly. Verify the wall can support the weight and is clear of obstructions before installing the sliding system.

Installation Guide

Putting Up the Upper Track
Find and mark the stud locations in the wall.
Level and line up the track with the marks.
Utilizing screws and anchors, fasten the track to the wall.
Putting up the Wall Panels
At the top of the panel, fasten mounting brackets.
Making sure the track is level and plumb, hang the panel onto it.
Putting the Rollers on
Fit the rollers to the panel's bottom.
If you want smooth functioning, adjust the rollers.
Locking the Panels
Fit a floor guide to secure the panel in position.

For easy mobility, include grips or handles.
Extras
Look for and caulk any gaps in the installation.
To be sure the sliding mechanism operates smoothly, test it.
Care and Repair Lubricating the rollers and cleaning the track are regular maintenance chores. In case the panel sticks or slides poorly, verify the alignment and make any roller adjustments.

Any room can benefit from and be made more attractive with a one-sided wall sliding system. You may take use of the advantages of this flexible system with the right tools and cautious installation.

GLUTE BRIDGE TO THE WALL

A glute, hamstring, and core muscle-stimulating variation of the traditional glute bridge exercise is the Glute Bridge to the Wall. People that need to strengthen their posterior chains and spend a lot of time sitting will find it especially beneficial.

Layout

Place a yoga mat or other soft surface on the floor up against a spotless wall.
Don comfortable clothing and take off your shoes to protect the wall.
Execution

Launching Position
Arms at your sides, lie on your back.
Keeping your knees bent at a 90-degree angle, walk your feet up the wall until they are flat on it, hip-width apart.
Thighs should be parallel to the ground.
The Lift
Activate your glutes and your core.
Raising your hips toward the ceiling, press your feet into the wall.
At the peak of the exercise, pause and make sure your body lines up from shoulders to knees.
The Slide
Regress your hips to where they were at first slowly.
For tension, keep your glutes just above the floor.
Reviews

Holding form and control throughout, do the exercise ten to fifteen repetitions.
For extra work, spend 20 to 30 seconds in the bridge position after finishing your repetitions.
Notes

For support of your lower back, keep your core tight.

Make that your glutes, not your back, propel the motion.

As you raise your hips, exhale and as you lower them, inhale.

Your glute strength and overall stability will be much increased if you include the Glute Bridge to the Wall in your routine. For best results from this workout, keep your attention on form and control.

LATERAL EXTENSION TO THE WALL

Exercises that work the muscles in the lower back and core, especially the obliques, include the Lateral Extension to the Wall. Strengthening lateral stability and strength is made easy with this exercise.

Assembly

Shoe-width apart, stand next to a wall.

An arm's length should separate your nearest body side from the wall.

Administration

Launching Position

Step firmly into the wall and lean your shoulder against it.

Press the hand of the arm nearest the wall against your hip.

The Extension

Holding your feet still, gently push your hips into the wall.

Your spine should make a "C" shape as your upper body slides laterally.

The Hold

Feeling the strain in your obliques, hold the end position for two to three seconds.

Watch that you move smoothly and under control.

The Return

Release slowly and take up your starting posture again.

Put in the necessary number of repetitions of the action.

Repertory

Ten to fifteen repetitions on each side are the goal.

For a well-rounded workout, do two to three sets.

Notes

To improve the involvement of your core muscles, move with calm and control.

As you stretch toward the wall, exhale, then inhale to get back to where you started.

Make sure you don't twist and that your back stays straight.

One easy but powerful exercise to improve lateral core stability and strength is the Lateral Extension to the Wall. It just needs a wall as additional equipment and may be quickly included into your training schedule.

ANGEL ON THE WALL

Known by another name, "Wall Angels," the "Angel on the Wall" exercise is a straightforward yet effective move designed to strengthen the muscles in the shoulders and upper back, improve posture, and increase shoulder range of motion.

Results

Increases mobility of the thoracic spine.
Fosters good posture.
Maybe lessen neck and back pain.
Excellent mobilization exercise before working out.
Layout

Lean against a wall, your back flat.
Slightly apart from the wall, feet should be shoulder-width apart.
Execution

Launching Position
Press your entire back—including the lower back's natural arch—against the wall.
Legs out in front of you, knees slightly bent.
Moving Arms
Press your triceps into the wall with your arms at your sides, level with your shoulders.
For a "goal post" form, rotate your arms upward so that your forearms and the backs of your hands both press against the wall.
Movement
Keeping your back and arms firmly against the wall, slowly raise your arms above your head.
Carry on until your elbows and shoulders are completely extended.
Once more, lower your arms until your triceps are parallel to the floor.
Reviews
Ten to fifteen repetitions of the exercise, keeping touch with the wall, should be completed.
A Common Error

Arching the back: To maximize the stretch and prevent strain, maintain a neutral spine.
Corrections and Variations

Shuffle your feet further away from the wall or place a little pillow behind your head for support if you find it hard to keep your head or hands on the wall.
Anyone wishing to improve their posture and shoulder health should definitely attempt this workout. Those who spend a lot of time at a desk or are attempting to warm up before a workout

are particularly benefiting from it. Better posture and less upper body strain may result from including this exercise in your regimen.

THUMB TO THE WALL

Those who are stiff or in discomfort from tendinitis or overuse may find the "Thumb to the Wall" exercise especially beneficial as it stretches and strengthens the muscles around the thumb.

Takeaways

More thumb movement.
Builds thumb muscles.
Helps to relieve overuse injury discomfort.
Layout

Approach a wall with the side of your afflicted arm closest to it.
For stability, space your feet shoulder width apart.
Execution

Opening Posture
Keeping your fingers pointing upward, press the palm of your injured hand against the wall at shoulder height.
Check that your thumb is free and not resting on the wall.
Extending
Holding your palm steady, lightly press the pad of your thumb against the wall.
Feel for a stretch into the wrist and along the inside of your thumb.
The Hold
Inhaling deeply to promote relaxation, hold the stretch for ten to fifteen seconds.
Keep your remainder of the body still and your posture perfect.
Agains
After releasing the stretch, do it two or three more times.
For the best effects, do this exercise several times during the day.
Notes

Thumbs should not be pushed into walls; the pressure should be minimal.
Should any pain arise, stop working out and see a doctor.
You can do this workout many times a day, particularly if you use your hands frequently for tasks like texting or typing.

Regular completion of the "Thumb to the Wall" exercise can improve thumb function and lessen pain. Particularly if you're prone to tendonitis or stiffness, this is an easy and effective way to maintain healthy thumbs.

Bonus

Practical Videos Workout

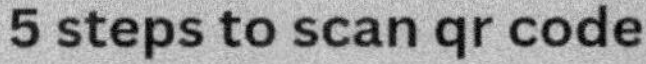

5 steps to scan qr code

1. Open your smartphone's camera app.

2. Point the camera at the QR code.

3. Allow the camera to focus and recognize the QR code.

4. Tap on the notification or follow the on-screen instructions to open the link or content.

5. If necessary, download any associated apps to access the content.

28 Days Workout Challenge Plan

Introducing Wall Pilates on Day 1

Warm the body up with some easy stretches first.
Discover Pilates breathing techniques.
Exercise fundamentally with wall squats and roll-downs.
Day Two: Core Activation

Emphasize using your core muscles.
Try wall plank and pelvic tilt movements against the wall.
Look at variations to put your core stability to the test.
Third Day: Developing the Upper Body

Build in tricep dips and wall push-ups.
Use the wall to align and support you.
Check your range of motion and form.
Day 4: Body Focus Lower

Work your legs with wall sits and single-leg wall bridges.
Stress exact alignment and control.
Get the thighs and glutes working.
Friday: Mobility and Flexibility

Add in dynamic stretches and mobility exercises.
Stretches including quadriceps and hamstrings can be supported by the wall.
Give each stretch your whole attention while you breathe and unwind.
On Day Six: Stability and Balance

Exercises that tax balance include single-leg stands against walls.
For increased stability, practice controlled, gradual motions.
Throughout, use your core to stay balanced.
Day 7: Rejoice and Heal

Spend a day relaxing and letting your body heal.
Give easy stretching or low-impact exercises like yoga or walking your full attention.
Day Eight: Fundamental Integration

Move both your upper and lower bodies while doing core workouts.
Take up wall toe taps and wall knee tucks.

Throughout every exercise, keep your core strong.
Day Nine: An Upper Body Challenge

Pick up the rigors of upper body workouts.
Try incline or decline push-ups, two variants of wall push-ups.
Give careful motions and the whole range of motion your attention.
Lower Body Burn on Day 10

Exercises for the lower body include wall lunges and squats.
For an increased difficulty, lengthen or intensify each workout.
As you increase strength and endurance, feel the muscles contracting.
Tenth Day: Fundamental Stability

Give stability workouts that tax the core your full attention.
Take up side plank variations or wall planks with leg raises.
Throughout every exercise, use your core muscles to keep your alignment correct.
Day 12: Length and Unwinding

Mix in some light stretching and relaxing exercises.
In stretches including spinal twists and chest openers, use the wall for support.
Give your full attention to inhaling deeply and releasing physical tension.
Day 13: Harmony in Progressions

Elevate balance workouts to increase stability difficulty.
Try wall balances with closed eyes or arm-movements during single-leg stands.
Balance requires control and attention.
Day 14: Relax and Revitalize

Give your body another day to heal completely.
Give self-care practices like foam rolling or meditation your whole attention.
Core Power on Day 15

Give dynamic core workouts that work every muscle in your body with your full attention.
Work in wall roll-ups and bicycle crunches against the wall.
All through, concentrate on controlled motions and core engagement.
Day 16: Upper Body Sturdiness

Longer sets or more repetitions will increase upper body muscle endurance.
Take up wall push-ups or lengthier holds on tricep dips.
Keep your breathing and form correct all the while.

Day 17: Weaker Body Systems

For strength building, up the ante on lower body workouts.
Test out wall squats with pulses or lengthier holds on single-leg wall bridges.
Stress using your glutes and thighs while pushing through your heels.
Day 18: Basic Control and Stability

Improve core stability by concentrating on controlled, slow motions.
Take up wall pikes or wall planks with shoulder taps.
Keep your breath calm and your core strong all the while.
Day 19: Striking a Balance

Work up the complexity of balance exercises.
Check out wall balances with knee lifts or single-leg stands with arm circles.
Give your full attention to each movement and maintain your presentness.
Twentieth Day: Mobility and Flexibility

Give your attention to deep stretching and increasing your flexibility.
Stretches including hip flexor or quad stretches can be supported by the wall.
Breathe deeply and let yourself unwind during every stretch.
Day 21: Soak and Think

Spend a day relaxing and considering your accomplishments thus far.
Honor your accomplishments and make fresh plans for the next week.
Day 22: Basic Endurance

Extend the sets of repetitions to build core muscular endurance.
Work out with plank grips or extended wall sit-ups.
Keep your breathing and form correct all the while.
Strengthening the Upper Body on Day 23

Make difficult exercises your main goal in developing upper body strength.
Take up tricep dips with raised feet or decline wall push-ups.
Emphasize using your chest and triceps while pushing through your palms.
Day 24: Lower Body Fortitude

Longer sets or higher repetitions will help lower body muscles become more resilient.
Take long holds on wall squats and wall lunges.
Keep your breathing and alignment correct all the while.
Day 25, Balance and Core Stability

For a full-body workout, mix stability and balance drills.
Exercises include single-leg stands with arm movements or wall planks with leg lifts.
Maintaining equilibrium throughout requires focus and control.
On Day 26, flexibility and relaxation

Emphasize deep stretching and relaxing methods.
For assistance when stretching your hamstrings or twisting your spine, use the wall.
Give your whole attention to inhaling deeply and releasing physical tension.
Day 27: Harmonious and Balanced

Pay attention to workouts that tax your coordination and balance.
Take up wall taps or arm-reaching single-leg stands.
Give each movement you do your whole attention.
Day 28: Joyful Reminiscence

Savor finishing the 28-day adventure and consider your development.
As you take stock of your progress, make fresh plans for the future.

Conclusion

Guided readers through the fundamental ideas and movements of Pilates with the additional support and stability of the wall, this is a transforming experience. With everything from easy exercises that promote mind-body connection to progressively developing strength, flexibility, and balance, this book enables readers to start a journey of self-discovery and overall health.

Readers who turn the pages become more physically strong as well as mentally resilient and peaceful inside. With each well described and illustrated practice, one moves closer to more energy and self-awareness.

Beyond simply a workout book, "Wall Pilates for Beginners" is a monument to the transformational potential and strength of tenacity. It exhorts readers to enjoy the ride, acknowledge each little accomplishment, and have faith in the natural wisdom of their bodies.

As they put the book down, readers come out as stewards of their own health and happiness as well as stronger, more adaptable people. They are prepared to face obstacles in life with elegance, composure, and a profound sense of inner power because they have gained newfound wisdom and confidence.